2000 Days Of Recipes: Discover Flavorful Galveston Delights On A Budget, Wallet-Friendly Dishes To Fuel Your Health And Well-Being, With A 30-Day Meal Plan

Wesley Hudson

Table of Contents

COPYRIGHT © 2023

CHAPTER ONE

Introduction to the Low Budget Galveston Diet

The Galveston Diet has gained significant popularity in recent years for its focus on women's health, particularly for those experiencing menopause. It emphasizes balanced nutrition, hormone regulation, and sustainable weight loss. However, adhering to a specific dietary regimen can sometimes be perceived as expensive. In this detailed exploration, we delve into the nuances of the Low Budget Galveston Diet, offering insights into its principles, benefits, and practical tips for grocery shopping on a budget.

Understanding the Galveston Diet Principles on a Budget

The Galveston Diet, developed by Dr. Mary Claire Haver, is designed to address the unique hormonal changes women undergo during menopause. It emphasizes the consumption of whole foods, healthy fats, lean proteins, and complex carbohydrates while minimizing processed foods, sugar, and refined carbohydrates. The diet aims to stabilize blood sugar levels, reduce inflammation, and support hormonal balance, leading to weight loss and improved overall health.

Transitioning the Galveston Diet principles to a budget-friendly approach requires strategic planning and informed choices. Here are some key strategies:

1. **Prioritize Whole Foods**: Whole foods, such as fruits, vegetables, whole grains, and legumes, form the foundation of the Galveston Diet. These foods are not only nutrient-dense but also tend to be more affordable than processed alternatives. Buying seasonal produce and opting for store brands can further reduce costs while maximizing nutritional value.

2. **Opt for Affordable Protein Sources**: Protein is essential for muscle maintenance, satiety, and hormone production. While animal proteins like chicken, turkey, and eggs are commonly recommended on the Galveston Diet, plant-based options like beans, lentils, tofu, and tempeh can be more budget-friendly alternatives. Buying in bulk or choosing frozen options can also lower expenses.

3. **Incorporate Healthy Fats**: Healthy fats, such as those found in avocados, nuts, seeds, and olive oil, play a crucial role in hormone regulation and satiety. While these items may seem expensive, they provide substantial nutritional benefits and can be used sparingly to stretch your budget. Consider purchasing in bulk or looking for sales to reduce costs.

4. **Minimize Processed Foods**: Processed foods, including sugary snacks, pre-packaged meals, and fast food, not only contribute to inflammation and hormonal imbalance but also strain your budget. By prioritizing whole, unprocessed foods, you can improve your health while saving money in the long run.

5. **Emphasize Meal Planning and Preparation**: Planning meals in advance and preparing them at home not only allows you to control ingredients and portion sizes but also helps minimize food waste and unnecessary spending. Utilize affordable staple ingredients, incorporate leftovers into future meals, and experiment with batch cooking to streamline your cooking process and maximize value.

By understanding and implementing these principles, you can adhere to the Galveston Diet while managing your budget effectively. With careful planning and smart choices, eating healthily doesn't have to break the bank.

Benefits of Following the Galveston Diet on a Budget

Following the Galveston Diet on a budget offers numerous benefits beyond just financial savings. Let's explore some of the advantages:

1. **Improved Health Outcomes**: The Galveston Diet prioritizes nutrient-dense foods that support hormonal balance, reduce inflammation, and stabilize blood sugar levels. By focusing on whole foods and minimizing processed items, you provide your body with the essential nutrients it needs to function optimally, leading to improved overall health and well-being.

2. **Weight Management**: One of the primary goals of the Galveston Diet is sustainable weight loss. By emphasizing lean proteins, healthy fats, and complex carbohydrates, while reducing sugar and refined carbohydrates, you can achieve and maintain a healthy weight more effectively. Additionally, the diet's focus on balancing hormones can help regulate appetite and prevent overeating, further supporting weight management goals.

3. **Increased Energy Levels**: The Galveston Diet promotes stable energy levels throughout the day by avoiding energy crashes associated with high-sugar and processed foods. By consuming nutrient-dense meals and snacks, you provide your body with a consistent source of fuel, resulting in sustained energy levels and improved productivity.

4. **Enhanced Mood and Mental Clarity**: Balanced nutrition is essential for brain health and cognitive function. The Galveston Diet's emphasis on whole foods rich in vitamins, minerals, and antioxidants can help support mental clarity,

focus, and mood stability. By nourishing your body with the right nutrients, you may experience reduced brain fog, improved mood, and enhanced overall cognitive function.

5. **Long-Term Cost Savings**: While there may be an initial adjustment period when transitioning to the Galveston Diet on a budget, the long-term cost savings can be significant. By prioritizing whole foods and minimizing expensive processed items, you not only save money on groceries but also reduce healthcare costs associated with poor dietary choices and related health conditions.

Overall, following the Galveston Diet on a budget offers a range of benefits that extend beyond financial savings, including improved health outcomes, weight management, increased energy levels, enhanced mood, and long-term cost savings. By prioritizing nutrient-dense foods and strategic meal planning, you can achieve your health and wellness goals without breaking the bank.

Tips for Grocery Shopping on a Budget

Grocery shopping on a budget requires careful planning, savvy shopping strategies, and a willingness to prioritize value over convenience. Here are some practical tips to help you stretch your dollars while adhering to the principles of the Galveston Diet:

1. **Create a Meal Plan**: Before heading to the grocery store, take the time to plan your meals for the week. Consider incorporating seasonal produce, utilizing ingredients you already have on hand, and preparing meals that can be repurposed for multiple dishes. Having a clear plan in place helps prevent impulse purchases and reduces food waste.

2. **Stick to a Shopping List**: Once you've established your meal plan, create a detailed shopping list based on the ingredients you need. Be sure to stick to your list while navigating the aisles to avoid unnecessary purchases. Consider organizing your list by category (e.g., produce, proteins, pantry staples) to streamline your shopping trip and minimize distractions.

3. **Shop the Perimeter**: The perimeter of the grocery store typically houses fresh produce, meats, dairy, and other whole foods, while the inner aisles contain more processed and packaged items. Focus your shopping efforts on the perimeter to prioritize nutrient-dense foods and minimize exposure to tempting but less nutritious options.

4. **Compare Prices and Brands**: Take the time to compare prices and brands to ensure you're getting the best value for your money. Consider opting for store brands or generic alternatives, which are often more affordable than name-brand products without sacrificing quality. Keep an eye out

for sales, discounts, and bulk packaging options to further maximize savings.

5. **Buy in Bulk and Freeze**: Purchasing items in bulk can often result in significant cost savings per unit. Look for bulk bins for grains, legumes, nuts, and spices, which allow you to purchase only the amount you need while avoiding unnecessary packaging. Additionally, consider buying extra quantities of perishable items when they're on sale and freezing them for future use to extend their shelf life and reduce waste.

6. **Utilize Coupons and Discounts**: Take advantage of coupons, loyalty programs, and digital discounts offered by grocery stores to further reduce your expenses. Many stores offer weekly specials and promotional deals on staple items, allowing you to stock up on essentials at a discounted price. Be sure to sign up for newsletters and download store apps to stay informed about current offers and savings opportunities.

7. **Consider Alternative Shopping Options**: In addition to traditional grocery stores, explore alternative shopping options such as farmers' markets, discount grocers, and online retailers. Farmers' markets often offer fresh, locally sourced produce at competitive prices, while discount grocers may carry affordable staple items and pantry

essentials. Online retailers may also offer bulk purchasing options and subscription services that can save you time and money in the long run.

By implementing these tips and strategies, you can navigate the grocery store with confidence, making informed choices that align with the principles of the Galveston Diet while staying within your budget. With a little planning and creativity, eating healthily on a budget is not only achievable but also rewarding in terms of both physical and financial well-being.

CHAPTER TWO

Affordable Breakfast Options

Breakfast is often considered the most important meal of the day, providing the fuel and nutrients needed to kickstart your morning. However, busy schedules and budget constraints can make it challenging to prepare nutritious breakfasts without breaking the bank. In this section, we explore affordable breakfast options that are not only budget-friendly but also delicious and easy to prepare.

Budget-Friendly Smoothie Recipes

Smoothies are a versatile and convenient breakfast option that can be customized to suit your taste preferences and nutritional needs. Here are some budget-friendly smoothie recipes that are packed with nutrients and flavor:

1. **Berry Blast Smoothie**:
   - Ingredients:
     - 1 cup frozen mixed berries
     - 1 banana (fresh or frozen)
     - 1/2 cup plain Greek yogurt
     - 1 tablespoon honey or maple syrup
     - 1 cup spinach or kale (optional)

- 1 cup water or unsweetened almond milk
- Instructions:

1. Combine all ingredients in a blender.

2. Blend until smooth and creamy.

3. Adjust sweetness to taste, adding more honey or maple syrup if desired.

4. Pour into a glass and enjoy immediately.

2. **Peanut Butter Banana Smoothie**:

- Ingredients:
  - 1 ripe banana
  - 2 tablespoons peanut butter
  - 1 tablespoon cocoa powder (optional)
  - 1 cup unsweetened almond milk
  - Ice cubes (optional)
- Instructions:

1. Peel the banana and break it into chunks.

2. Place banana chunks, peanut butter, cocoa powder (if using), almond milk, and ice cubes (if desired) in a blender.

3. Blend until smooth and creamy.

4.   Pour into a glass and serve.

3. **Green Goddess Smoothie**:

- Ingredients:

    - 1/2 cup frozen mango chunks

    - 1/2 cup frozen pineapple chunks

    - 1 cup spinach or kale

    - 1/2 avocado

    - 1 tablespoon chia seeds

    - 1 cup coconut water

- Instructions:

1.   Combine all ingredients in a blender.

2.   Blend until smooth and creamy.

3.   Add more coconut water if necessary to reach desired consistency.

4.   Pour into a glass and enjoy.

These budget-friendly smoothie recipes are not only delicious but also packed with vitamins, minerals, and antioxidants to fuel your day without breaking the bank.

Simple Overnight Oats Variations

Overnight oats are a popular breakfast option that can be prepared in advance and customized with various toppings and flavors. Here are some simple overnight oats variations that are perfect for budget-conscious individuals:

1. **Classic Overnight Oats**:

    - Ingredients:

        - 1/2 cup rolled oats

        - 1/2 cup milk (dairy or plant-based)

        - 1/2 cup Greek yogurt

        - 1 tablespoon chia seeds (optional)

        - 1 tablespoon honey or maple syrup (optional)

    - Instructions:

1.   In a mason jar or container, combine rolled oats, milk, Greek yogurt, chia seeds (if using), and honey or maple syrup (if desired).

2.   Stir well to combine.

3.   Cover and refrigerate overnight or for at least 4 hours.

4.   In the morning, give the oats a good stir, add your favorite toppings, and enjoy cold or warmed up.

2. **Banana Nut Overnight Oats**:

- Ingredients:

    - 1/2 cup rolled oats

    - 1/2 cup milk (dairy or plant-based)

    - 1/2 ripe banana, mashed

    - 1 tablespoon chopped nuts (such as almonds, walnuts, or pecans)

    - 1/2 teaspoon cinnamon

- Instructions:

1. In a mason jar or container, combine rolled oats, milk, mashed banana, chopped nuts, and cinnamon.

2. Stir well to combine.

3. Cover and refrigerate overnight or for at least 4 hours.

4. In the morning, give the oats a good stir, add additional toppings if desired, and enjoy.

3. **Apple Cinnamon Overnight Oats**:

- Ingredients:

    - 1/2 cup rolled oats

    - 1/2 cup milk (dairy or plant-based)

- 1/2 apple, diced

- 1 tablespoon raisins or dried cranberries

- 1/2 teaspoon cinnamon

- Instructions:

1. In a mason jar or container, combine rolled oats, milk, diced apple, raisins or dried cranberries, and cinnamon.

2. Stir well to combine.

3. Cover and refrigerate overnight or for at least 4 hours.

4. In the morning, give the oats a good stir, add a drizzle of honey or maple syrup if desired, and enjoy.

These simple overnight oats variations are not only affordable but also versatile, allowing you to customize them with your favorite ingredients and flavors for a delicious and nutritious breakfast.

DIY Breakfast Bars and Bites

Homemade breakfast bars and bites are a convenient grab-and-go option that can be made in advance and enjoyed throughout the week. Here are some DIY recipes for budget-friendly breakfast bars and bites:

1. **No-Bake Peanut Butter Oat Bars**:

- Ingredients:

- 1 cup rolled oats

- 1/2 cup peanut butter

- 1/4 cup honey or maple syrup

- 1/4 cup chopped nuts or seeds (such as almonds, walnuts, or sunflower seeds)

- 1/4 cup dried fruit (such as raisins, cranberries, or apricots)

- Instructions:

1. In a mixing bowl, combine rolled oats, peanut butter, honey or maple syrup, chopped nuts or seeds, and dried fruit.

2. Stir until well combined and the mixture holds together.

3. Press the mixture into a lined baking dish or pan, using a spatula or your hands to flatten it evenly.

4. Refrigerate for at least 1 hour to set, then cut into bars or squares.

5. Store in an airtight container in the refrigerator for up to one week.

2. **Homemade Granola Bars**:

- Ingredients:

  - 2 cups rolled oats

- 1/2 cup almond butter or peanut butter

- 1/4 cup honey or maple syrup

- 1/4 cup chopped nuts or seeds (such as almonds, pecans, or pumpkin seeds)

- 1/4 cup dried fruit (such as raisins, cranberries, or chopped dates)

- 1/4 cup chocolate chips (optional)

- Instructions:

1. Preheat your oven to 350°F (175°C) and line a baking dish or pan with parchment paper.

2. In a mixing bowl, combine rolled oats, almond butter or peanut butter, honey or maple syrup, chopped nuts or seeds, dried fruit, and chocolate chips (if using).

3. Stir until well combined and the mixture holds together.

4. Press the mixture into the prepared baking dish or pan, using a spatula or your hands to flatten it evenly.

5. Bake for 15-20 minutes or until golden brown and set.

6. Allow to cool completely before cutting into bars.

7. Store in an airtight container at room temperature for up to one week.

3. **Energy Bites**:

- Ingredients:
    - 1 cup rolled oats
    - 1/2 cup nut butter (such as almond butter, peanut butter, or cashew butter)
    - 1/4 cup honey or maple syrup
    - 1/4 cup shredded coconut
    - 1/4 cup mini chocolate chips
    - 1 teaspoon vanilla extract
- Instructions:

1. In a mixing bowl, combine rolled oats, nut butter, honey or maple syrup, shredded coconut, chocolate chips, and vanilla extract.

2. Stir until well combined and the mixture holds together.

3. Using your hands, roll the mixture into small bite-sized balls.

4. Place the energy bites on a lined baking sheet and refrigerate for at least 30 minutes to set.

5. Once set, transfer the energy bites to an airtight container and store in the refrigerator for up to one week.

These DIY breakfast bars and bites are not only cost-effective but also customizable, allowing you to tailor them to your taste preferences and dietary needs. Prepare a batch at the beginning of the week for a convenient and nutritious breakfast option on the go.

CHAPTER THREE

Budget-Friendly Lunch Ideas

Lunchtime offers an opportunity to refuel and recharge for the rest of the day. However, finding affordable yet satisfying options can be challenging. In this section, we explore budget-friendly lunch ideas that are both nutritious and wallet-friendly.

Frugal Salad Creations with Seasonal Produce

Salads are a versatile and nutrient-rich option for lunch, especially when prepared with seasonal produce that tends to be more affordable. Here are some frugal salad creations to inspire your lunchtime meals:

1. **Seasonal Veggie Salad**:

    - Ingredients:

        - Mixed greens (such as spinach, kale, or lettuce)

        - Seasonal vegetables (such as tomatoes, cucumbers, bell peppers, carrots, and radishes)

        - Protein source (such as grilled chicken, hard-boiled eggs, chickpeas, or tofu)

        - Optional toppings (such as nuts, seeds, cheese, or dried fruit)

    - Dressing:

- Olive oil

- Balsamic vinegar

- Dijon mustard

- Lemon juice

- Salt and pepper to taste

- Instructions:

1. Wash and chop the mixed greens and seasonal vegetables.

2. Add the vegetables to a large bowl along with your choice of protein source.

3. Top with optional toppings such as nuts, seeds, cheese, or dried fruit.

4. In a small jar, combine the dressing ingredients and shake well to emulsify.

5. Drizzle the dressing over the salad just before serving and toss to coat evenly.

2. **Quinoa and Roasted Vegetable Salad**:

- Ingredients:

- Cooked quinoa

- Seasonal vegetables (such as zucchini, eggplant, cherry tomatoes, and onions)

- Olive oil

  - Salt and pepper

  - Fresh herbs (such as parsley, basil, or thyme)

  - Feta cheese or goat cheese (optional)

- Dressing:

  - Olive oil

  - Lemon juice

  - Dijon mustard

  - Honey or maple syrup

  - Salt and pepper to taste

- Instructions:

1. Preheat the oven to 400°F (200°C).

2. Toss the seasonal vegetables with olive oil, salt, and pepper on a baking sheet.

3. Roast in the preheated oven for 20-25 minutes or until tender and caramelized.

4. In a large bowl, combine the cooked quinoa, roasted vegetables, and fresh herbs.

5. Crumble feta cheese or goat cheese over the salad if desired.

6.   In a small jar, combine the dressing ingredients and shake well to emulsify.

7.   Drizzle the dressing over the salad just before serving and toss to coat evenly.

3. **Bean and Corn Salad**:

- Ingredients:

    - Canned beans (such as black beans, kidney beans, or chickpeas)

    - Corn kernels (fresh, frozen, or canned)

    - Bell peppers (any color), diced

    - Red onion, finely chopped

    - Fresh cilantro, chopped

    - Lime juice

    - Olive oil

    - Salt and pepper to taste

- Instructions:

1.   Rinse and drain the canned beans and corn kernels (if using canned).

2.   In a large bowl, combine the beans, corn, diced bell peppers, chopped red onion, and chopped cilantro.

3.   Drizzle with lime juice and olive oil, and season with salt and pepper to taste.

4.   Toss the salad gently to combine all the ingredients.

5.   Let the flavors marinate for at least 15 minutes before serving.

These frugal salad creations with seasonal produce are not only budget-friendly but also packed with vitamins, minerals, and fiber to keep you feeling satisfied and energized throughout the day.

Budget-Friendly Soup and Stew Recipes

Soups and stews are hearty and comforting lunch options that can be made in large batches and enjoyed throughout the week. Here are some budget-friendly recipes to warm up your lunchtime:

1. **Vegetable and Lentil Soup:**

   - Ingredients:

     - 1 tablespoon olive oil

     - 1 onion, diced

     - 2 carrots, diced

     - 2 celery stalks, diced

     - 2 cloves garlic, minced

- 1 cup dried green or brown lentils, rinsed and drained

- 4 cups vegetable broth

- 1 can diced tomatoes

- 2 teaspoons dried thyme

- Salt and pepper to taste

- Instructions:

1. In a large pot, heat olive oil over medium heat.

2. Add diced onion, carrots, and celery, and sauté until softened, about 5 minutes.

3. Add minced garlic and cook for an additional minute.

4. Stir in dried lentils, vegetable broth, diced tomatoes, and dried thyme.

5. Bring the soup to a boil, then reduce heat and simmer for 20-25 minutes, or until the lentils are tender.

6. Season with salt and pepper to taste before serving.

2. **Chicken and Vegetable Stew**:

- Ingredients:

- 1 tablespoon olive oil

- 1 onion, diced

- 2 carrots, diced

- 2 celery stalks, diced

- 2 cloves garlic, minced

- 1 pound boneless, skinless chicken thighs, cut into bite-sized pieces

- 4 cups chicken broth

- 1 can diced tomatoes

- 2 teaspoons dried thyme

- Salt and pepper to taste

- Instructions:

1. In a large pot, heat olive oil over medium heat.

2. Add diced onion, carrots, and celery, and sauté until softened, about 5 minutes.

3. Add minced garlic and cook for an additional minute.

4. Add the diced chicken thighs to the pot and cook until browned on all sides.

5. Stir in chicken broth, diced tomatoes, and dried thyme.

6.   Bring the stew to a boil, then reduce heat and simmer for 20-25 minutes, or until the chicken is cooked through and the vegetables are tender.

7.   Season with salt and pepper to taste before serving.

3. **Bean and Vegetable Chili**:

- Ingredients:

    - 1 tablespoon olive oil

    - 1 onion, diced

    - 2 bell peppers (any color), diced

    - 2 cloves garlic, minced

    - 2 teaspoons chili powder

    - 1 teaspoon cumin

    - 1 can black beans, drained and rinsed

    - 1 can kidney beans, drained and rinsed

    - 1 can diced tomatoes

    - 2 cups vegetable broth

    - Salt and pepper to taste

- Instructions:

1.   In a large pot, heat olive oil over medium heat.

2.   Add diced onion and bell peppers, and sauté until softened, about 5 minutes.

3.   Add minced garlic, chili powder, and cumin, and cook for an additional minute.

4.   Stir in black beans, kidney beans, diced tomatoes, and vegetable broth.

5.   Bring the chili to a boil, then reduce heat and simmer for 20-25 minutes, stirring occasionally.

6.   Season with salt and pepper to taste before serving.

These budget-friendly soup and stew recipes are not only delicious and satisfying but also perfect for batch cooking and meal prep, allowing you to enjoy homemade lunches throughout the week without breaking the bank.

Sandwiches and Wraps on a Shoestring Budget

Sandwiches and wraps are classic lunchtime staples that can be customized with an array of ingredients to suit your taste and budget. Here are some wallet-friendly ideas to inspire your next sandwich or wrap creation:

1. **Classic Veggie Sandwich**:

   - Ingredients:

     - Whole grain bread slices

- Hummus or avocado spread

- Sliced cucumber

- Sliced tomato

- Thinly sliced red onion

- Leafy greens (such as lettuce or spinach)

- Instructions:

1. Spread hummus or mashed avocado on one slice of whole grain bread.

2. Layer cucumber slices, tomato slices, thinly sliced red onion, and leafy greens on top.

3. Top with another slice of bread and press gently to secure the sandwich.

4. Cut the sandwich in half diagonally and serve.

2. **Turkey and Cheese Wrap**:

- Ingredients:

    - Whole wheat tortilla

    - Sliced turkey breast

    - Sliced cheese (such as cheddar or Swiss)

    - Thinly sliced cucumber

- Shredded carrots

- Dijon mustard or mayonnaise

- Instructions:

1. Lay a whole wheat tortilla flat on a clean surface.

2. Spread Dijon mustard or mayonnaise evenly over the tortilla.

3. Layer sliced turkey breast, sliced cheese, thinly sliced cucumber, and shredded carrots down the center of the tortilla.

4. Roll up the tortilla tightly, tucking in the sides as you go.

5. Slice the wrap in half diagonally and serve.

3. **Tuna Salad Sandwich**:

- Ingredients:

  - Whole grain bread slices

  - Canned tuna, drained

  - Greek yogurt or mayonnaise

  - Dijon mustard

  - Chopped celery

  - Chopped red onion

  - Salt and pepper to taste

- Instructions:

1.   In a mixing bowl, combine canned tuna, Greek yogurt or mayonnaise, Dijon mustard, chopped celery, and chopped red onion.

2.   Stir until well combined, and season with salt and pepper to taste.

3.   Spread the tuna salad mixture evenly onto one slice of whole grain bread.

4.   Top with another slice of bread and press gently to secure the sandwich.

5.   Cut the sandwich in half diagonally and serve.

These sandwiches and wraps on a shoestring budget are not only affordable but also versatile, allowing you to customize them with your favorite ingredients and flavors for a satisfying lunchtime meal without breaking the bank.

CHAPTER FOUR

Economical Snack Solutions

Snacks play an essential role in maintaining energy levels and staving off hunger between meals. However, purchasing pre-packaged snacks can quickly add up in terms of cost. In this section, we explore economical snack solutions that are not only budget-friendly but also delicious and nutritious.

Low-Cost Nut and Seed Mixes

Nuts and seeds are nutrient-dense snacks packed with protein, healthy fats, fiber, vitamins, and minerals. Creating your own nut and seed mixes at home allows you to customize flavors while saving money. Here are some ideas for low-cost nut and seed mixes:

1. **Basic Nut Mix**:

   - Ingredients:

     - Almonds

     - Walnuts

     - Cashews

     - Peanuts

     - Pecans

   - Instructions:

1.   Combine equal parts of almonds, walnuts, cashews, peanuts, and pecans in a large bowl.

2.   Toss the nuts together until well mixed.

3.   Store the nut mix in an airtight container or portion it into individual snack bags for easy grab-and-go convenience.

2. **Seed and Fruit Mix**:

- Ingredients:
    - Pumpkin seeds (pepitas)
    - Sunflower seeds
    - Dried cranberries
    - Raisins
    - Dried apricots, chopped
- Instructions:

1.   In a large bowl, combine equal parts pumpkin seeds, sunflower seeds, dried cranberries, raisins, and chopped dried apricots.

2.   Toss the seeds and fruits together until well mixed.

3.   Store the seed and fruit mix in an airtight container or portion it into individual snack bags for easy snacking on the go.

3. **Spiced Nut Mix**:

- Ingredients:

  - Almonds

  - Pecans

  - Cashews

  - Olive oil

  - Salt

  - Ground cinnamon

  - Ground cumin

  - Ground paprika

  - Ground cayenne pepper (optional for heat)

- Instructions:

1. Preheat the oven to 300°F (150°C).

2. In a large bowl, toss equal parts almonds, pecans, and cashews with a drizzle of olive oil and a sprinkle of salt.

3. In a small bowl, mix together ground cinnamon, ground cumin, ground paprika, and ground cayenne pepper (if using).

4. Sprinkle the spice mixture over the nuts and toss until evenly coated.

5.   Spread the seasoned nuts in a single layer on a baking sheet lined with parchment paper.

6.   Bake for 15-20 minutes, stirring halfway through, until the nuts are golden and fragrant.

7.   Allow the spiced nut mix to cool completely before transferring it to an airtight container for storage.

These low-cost nut and seed mixes are not only delicious and satisfying but also provide a healthy dose of essential nutrients to keep you fueled throughout the day.

Homemade Popcorn and Veggie Chips

Popcorn and veggie chips are crunchy, satisfying snacks that can be made at home for a fraction of the cost of store-bought alternatives. Here are some ideas for homemade popcorn and veggie chips:

1. **Air-Popped Popcorn**:

   - Ingredients:

     - Popcorn kernels

     - Olive oil or melted butter (optional)

     - Salt

   - Instructions:

1.   Place a handful of popcorn kernels in an air popper.

2.   Turn on the air popper and let it pop the kernels until they're all popped.

3.   Transfer the popped popcorn to a large bowl.

4.   Drizzle with olive oil or melted butter (if using) and sprinkle with salt to taste.

5.   Toss the popcorn until evenly coated with the oil and salt.

6.   Enjoy immediately or store in an airtight container for later snacking.

2. **Baked Veggie Chips**:

- Ingredients:

    - Assorted vegetables (such as sweet potatoes, beets, carrots, zucchini, or kale)

    - Olive oil

    - Salt and pepper

- Instructions:

1.   Preheat the oven to 375°F (190°C).

2.   Wash and peel the vegetables, if necessary, and slice them thinly using a mandoline or sharp knife.

3.   Place the sliced vegetables in a single layer on baking sheets lined with parchment paper.

4.   Drizzle the vegetables with olive oil and sprinkle with salt and pepper.

5.   Bake in the preheated oven for 15-20 minutes, flipping halfway through, until the chips are crisp and golden brown.

6.   Allow the veggie chips to cool completely before storing them in an airtight container.

3. **Spicy Kale Chips**:

- Ingredients:

    - Fresh kale leaves, stems removed and torn into bite-sized pieces

    - Olive oil

    - Salt

    - Ground cayenne pepper

- Instructions:

1.   Preheat the oven to 300°F (150°C).

2.   Place the torn kale leaves in a large bowl and drizzle with olive oil.

3.   Sprinkle with salt and ground cayenne pepper to taste.

4.   Toss the kale leaves until evenly coated with the oil and seasoning.

5.   Spread the seasoned kale leaves in a single layer on baking sheets lined with parchment paper.

6.   Bake in the preheated oven for 10-15 minutes, or until the kale chips are crispy and slightly golden.

7.   Allow the kale chips to cool completely before storing them in an airtight container.

These homemade popcorn and veggie chips are not only budget-friendly but also healthier alternatives to store-bought snacks, allowing you to indulge in crunchy goodness without breaking the bank.

Budget-Friendly Fruit Snacks and Dips

Fruits are nature's candy, offering sweetness and nutrition in one convenient package. Pairing fruits with budget-friendly dips adds flavor and variety to your snack routine. Here are some ideas for budget-friendly fruit snacks and dips:

1. **Apple Slices with Peanut Butter**:

   - Ingredients:

     - Apples, sliced

     - Peanut butter (or almond butter for a variation)

   - Instructions:

1.   Wash and slice apples into wedges or rounds, removing any seeds or stems.

2.   Spread peanut butter on one side of each apple slice.

3.   Arrange the apple slices on a plate and serve immediately.

2. **Banana Slices with Greek Yogurt**:

- Ingredients:

    - Bananas, sliced

    - Greek yogurt

- Instructions:

1.   Peel and slice bananas into rounds.

2.   Dip each banana slice into Greek yogurt, coating it evenly.

3.   Place the yogurt-coated banana slices on a parchment-lined baking sheet.

4.   Freeze for 1-2 hours until the yogurt is set.

5.   Serve immediately or transfer to an airtight container and store in the freezer for later snacking.

3. **Mixed Fruit Skewers with Honey Yogurt Dip**:

- Ingredients:

- Assorted fruits (such as strawberries, grapes, pineapple chunks, and melon cubes)

- Wooden skewers

- Greek yogurt

- Honey

- Instructions:

1. Wash and prepare the fruits as needed, cutting them into bite-sized pieces.

2. Thread the fruit pieces onto wooden skewers, alternating colors and shapes.

3. In a small bowl, mix Greek yogurt with honey to taste.

4. Serve the mixed fruit skewers with the honey yogurt dip on the side for dipping.

These budget-friendly fruit snacks and dips are not only delicious and satisfying but also provide a refreshing burst of vitamins, minerals, and antioxidants to keep you feeling energized throughout the day. Experiment with different fruit combinations and dip flavors to keep your snack time interesting and enjoyable.

CHAPTER FIVE

Dinner on a Dime

When it comes to preparing dinner on a budget, creativity and resourcefulness are key. In this section, we explore cost-effective dinner ideas that are both delicious and wallet-friendly.

Budget-Friendly One-Pot Meals

One-pot meals are a budget-conscious cook's best friend. They require minimal ingredients, use up leftovers, and require less cleanup. Here are some ideas for budget-friendly one-pot meals:

1. **Vegetable Stir-Fry**:

   - Ingredients:

     - Assorted vegetables (such as bell peppers, broccoli, carrots, snap peas, and mushrooms), chopped

     - Protein source (such as tofu, chicken, shrimp, or beef), diced

     - Cooking oil (such as olive oil or sesame oil)

     - Soy sauce

     - Garlic, minced

     - Ginger, grated (optional)

- Cooked rice or noodles (optional, for serving)

- Instructions:

1. Heat oil in a large skillet or wok over medium-high heat.

2. Add minced garlic and grated ginger (if using) to the skillet and cook for 1 minute until fragrant.

3. Add chopped vegetables to the skillet and cook until tender-crisp, stirring frequently.

4. Push the vegetables to one side of the skillet and add diced protein source to the other side.

5. Cook the protein until browned and cooked through, then combine with the vegetables.

6. Drizzle soy sauce over the stir-fry and toss to coat evenly.

7. Serve the vegetable stir-fry as is or over cooked rice or noodles, if desired.

2. **Chili Con Carne**:

- Ingredients:

  - Ground beef

  - Onion, diced

  - Bell peppers, diced

  - Canned kidney beans, drained and rinsed

- Canned diced tomatoes

- Tomato paste

- Chili powder

- Cumin

- Salt and pepper

- Instructions:

1. In a large pot or Dutch oven, brown ground beef over medium heat, breaking it up with a spoon.

2. Add diced onion and bell peppers to the pot and cook until softened.

3. Stir in canned kidney beans, canned diced tomatoes, tomato paste, chili powder, cumin, salt, and pepper.

4. Bring the chili to a simmer and cook for 20-30 minutes, stirring occasionally, until the flavors meld together and the chili thickens.

5. Serve the chili hot, garnished with your favorite toppings such as shredded cheese, sour cream, and chopped green onions.

3. **One-Pot Pasta Primavera**:

- Ingredients:

- Pasta (such as penne, fusilli, or spaghetti)

- Assorted vegetables (such as zucchini, cherry tomatoes, bell peppers, and spinach), chopped

- Garlic, minced

- Olive oil

- Vegetable or chicken broth

- Grated Parmesan cheese (optional)

- Instructions:

1. In a large pot or skillet, heat olive oil over medium heat.

2. Add minced garlic to the pot and cook for 1 minute until fragrant.

3. Add chopped vegetables to the pot and sauté until tender.

4. Pour vegetable or chicken broth into the pot and bring to a boil.

5. Add pasta to the pot and cook according to package instructions until al dente.

6. Once the pasta is cooked, remove the pot from heat and stir in grated Parmesan cheese (if using).

7. Serve the one-pot pasta primavera hot, garnished with additional Parmesan cheese if desired.

These budget-friendly one-pot meals are not only convenient and easy to prepare but also packed with flavor and nutrition, making them perfect for satisfying weeknight dinners without breaking the bank.

Versatile Rice and Bean Dishes

Rice and beans are pantry staples that form the basis of many affordable and satisfying meals. Here are some ideas for versatile rice and bean dishes:

1. **Bean and Rice Burrito Bowl**:

   - Ingredients:
     - Cooked rice (such as white rice, brown rice, or quinoa)
     - Canned black beans, drained and rinsed
     - Corn kernels (fresh, frozen, or canned)
     - Salsa
     - Avocado, diced
     - Fresh cilantro, chopped
     - Lime wedges
   - Instructions:

1. Divide cooked rice among serving bowls.

2.   Top the rice with canned black beans, corn kernels, salsa, diced avocado, and chopped fresh cilantro.

3.   Squeeze lime wedges over the burrito bowls before serving.

  2. **Vegetable Fried Rice**:

- Ingredients:

    - Cooked rice (preferably day-old rice)

    - Assorted vegetables (such as carrots, peas, corn, bell peppers, and broccoli), diced

    - Onion, diced

    - Garlic, minced

    - Eggs, beaten

    - Soy sauce

    - Sesame oil

    - Green onions, chopped (optional)

- Instructions:

1.   Heat oil in a large skillet or wok over medium-high heat.

2.   Add diced onion and minced garlic to the skillet and cook until softened.

3.   Push the onion and garlic to one side of the skillet and pour beaten eggs into the other side.

4.   Scramble the eggs until cooked through, then combine with the onion and garlic.

5.   Add diced vegetables to the skillet and stir-fry until tender.

6.   Add cooked rice to the skillet along with soy sauce and sesame oil to taste.

7.   Stir-fry everything together until well combined and heated through.

8.   Garnish with chopped green onions before serving.

3. **Red Beans and Rice**:

- Ingredients:
    - Cooked rice (such as white rice or brown rice)
    - Canned red kidney beans, drained and rinsed
    - Onion, diced
    - Bell pepper, diced
    - Celery, diced
    - Garlic, minced
    - Cajun seasoning

- Chicken or vegetable broth

- Green onions, chopped (optional)

- Instructions:

1. Heat oil in a large pot or skillet over medium heat.

2. Add diced onion, bell pepper, celery, and minced garlic to the pot and cook until softened.

3. Stir in Cajun seasoning to taste.

4. Add canned red kidney beans and chicken or vegetable broth to the pot.

5. Bring the mixture to a simmer and cook for 15-20 minutes, stirring occasionally, until the flavors meld together and the beans are heated through.

6. Serve the red beans and rice hot, garnished with chopped green onions if desired.

These versatile rice and bean dishes are not only economical and filling but also customizable, allowing you to use up whatever ingredients you have on hand to create delicious and satisfying meals for the whole family.

Budget-Friendly Pasta and Sauce Combos

Pasta is a pantry staple that can be transformed into countless budget-friendly meals with the addition of simple sauces and ingredients. Here are some ideas for budget-friendly pasta and sauce combos:

1. **Spaghetti Aglio e Olio**:

  - Ingredients:

    - Spaghetti pasta

    - Garlic, thinly sliced

    - Red pepper flakes

    - Olive oil

    - Fresh parsley, chopped

  - Instructions:

1.   Cook spaghetti pasta according to package instructions until al dente.

2.   While the pasta is cooking, heat olive oil in a large skillet over medium heat.

3.   Add thinly sliced garlic and red pepper flakes to the skillet and cook until the garlic is golden brown and fragrant.

4.   Drain the cooked pasta and add it to the skillet, tossing to coat in the garlic-infused oil.

5.   Stir in chopped fresh parsley and season with salt to taste.

6.   Serve the spaghetti aglio e olio hot, garnished with additional parsley if desired.

2. **Pasta with Marinara Sauce**:

- Ingredients:

  - Pasta of your choice (such as spaghetti, penne, or farfalle)

  - Canned diced tomatoes

  - Tomato paste

  - Onion, diced

  - Garlic, minced

  - Italian seasoning (such as dried basil, oregano, and thyme)

  - Olive oil

  - Salt and pepper

- Instructions:

1.   Cook pasta according to package instructions until al dente.

2.   While the pasta is cooking, heat olive oil in a large skillet over medium heat.

3.   Add diced onion and minced garlic to the skillet and cook until softened.

4.   Stir in canned diced tomatoes, tomato paste, and Italian seasoning.

5.   Simmer the marinara sauce for 10-15 minutes, stirring occasionally, until thickened.

6.   Season with salt and pepper to taste.

7.   Serve the pasta with marinara sauce hot, garnished with grated Parmesan cheese if desired.

3. **Creamy Garlic Parmesan Pasta**:

- Ingredients:
    - Pasta of your choice (such as fettuccine or linguine)
    - Garlic, minced
    - Butter
    - All-purpose flour
    - Milk
    - Grated Parmesan cheese
    - Salt and pepper
    - Fresh parsley, chopped (optional)
- Instructions:

1.   Cook pasta according to package instructions until al dente.

2.   While the pasta is cooking, melt butter in a large skillet over medium heat.

3.   Add minced garlic to the skillet and cook until fragrant.

4.   Stir in all-purpose flour to form a roux, cooking for 1-2 minutes until lightly golden.

5.   Gradually whisk in milk, stirring constantly, until the sauce thickens.

6.   Stir in grated Parmesan cheese until melted and smooth.

7.   Season the sauce with salt and pepper to taste.

8.   Drain the cooked pasta and toss it in the creamy garlic Parmesan sauce until evenly coated.

9.   Serve the pasta hot, garnished with chopped fresh parsley if desired.

These budget-friendly pasta and sauce combos are not only simple and delicious but also versatile, allowing you to customize them with your favorite ingredients and flavors for a satisfying dinner without breaking the bank.

CHAPTER SIX

Thrifty Side Dishes

When planning a meal on a budget, side dishes can often be overlooked. However, with a little creativity and resourcefulness, you can create delicious and satisfying side dishes that complement your main course without breaking the bank. In this section, we explore thrifty side dish ideas that are both affordable and flavorful.

Budget-Friendly Roasted Vegetables

Roasting vegetables is a simple and economical way to enhance their natural flavors and textures. Here are some ideas for budget-friendly roasted vegetable side dishes:

1. **Mixed Roasted Vegetables**:

   - Ingredients:

     - Assorted vegetables (such as carrots, potatoes, sweet potatoes, onions, bell peppers, and zucchini), chopped into bite-sized pieces

     - Olive oil

     - Salt and pepper

     - Optional herbs and spices (such as garlic powder, paprika, or dried herbs)

- Instructions:

1. Preheat the oven to 400°F (200°C).

2. Spread chopped vegetables in a single layer on a baking sheet lined with parchment paper.

3. Drizzle olive oil over the vegetables and season with salt, pepper, and any desired herbs and spices.

4. Toss the vegetables until evenly coated with oil and seasonings.

5. Roast in the preheated oven for 25-30 minutes, stirring halfway through, until the vegetables are tender and caramelized.

6. Serve the roasted vegetables hot as a flavorful and nutritious side dish.

2. **Parmesan Roasted Broccoli**:

- Ingredients:

  - Fresh broccoli florets

  - Olive oil

  - Grated Parmesan cheese

  - Salt and pepper

- Instructions:

1. Preheat the oven to 425°F (220°C).

2.   Toss broccoli florets with olive oil until evenly coated.

3.   Spread the broccoli florets in a single layer on a baking sheet lined with parchment paper.

4.   Sprinkle grated Parmesan cheese over the broccoli and season with salt and pepper to taste.

5.   Roast in the preheated oven for 15-20 minutes, or until the broccoli is tender and the edges are crispy.

6.   Serve the Parmesan roasted broccoli hot as a delicious and nutritious side dish.

3. **Honey Glazed Carrots**:

- Ingredients:
    - Carrots, peeled and sliced into rounds
    - Olive oil
    - Honey
    - Salt and pepper
- Instructions:

1.   Preheat the oven to 400°F (200°C).

2.   Toss carrot rounds with olive oil until evenly coated.

3.   Spread the carrot rounds in a single layer on a baking sheet lined with parchment paper.

4.   Drizzle honey over the carrots and season with salt and pepper to taste.

5.   Roast in the preheated oven for 20-25 minutes, stirring halfway through, until the carrots are tender and caramelized.

6.   Serve the honey glazed carrots hot as a sweet and savory side dish.

These budget-friendly roasted vegetable side dishes are not only delicious and satisfying but also packed with vitamins, minerals, and fiber, making them a nutritious addition to any meal.

Affordable Side Salads with Simple Dressings

Side salads are a versatile and refreshing addition to any meal, offering a burst of freshness and flavor. Here are some ideas for affordable side salads with simple dressings:

1. **Classic Garden Salad**:

- Ingredients:

    - Mixed salad greens (such as lettuce, spinach, and arugula)

    - Cherry tomatoes, halved

    - Cucumber, sliced

    - Red onion, thinly sliced

- Balsamic vinaigrette dressing (olive oil, balsamic vinegar, Dijon mustard, salt, and pepper)

- Instructions:

1. In a large bowl, combine mixed salad greens, cherry tomatoes, cucumber slices, and thinly sliced red onion.

2. Drizzle with balsamic vinaigrette dressing and toss until evenly coated.

3. Serve the classic garden salad cold as a refreshing and nutritious side dish.

2. **Coleslaw with Creamy Dressing**:

- Ingredients:

  - Shredded cabbage (green and/or red)

  - Carrots, grated

  - Green onions, thinly sliced

  - Mayonnaise

  - Apple cider vinegar

  - Honey or sugar

  - Salt and pepper

- Instructions:

1.   In a large bowl, combine shredded cabbage, grated carrots, and thinly sliced green onions.

2.   In a small bowl, whisk together mayonnaise, apple cider vinegar, honey or sugar, salt, and pepper to taste.

3.   Pour the creamy dressing over the coleslaw and toss until evenly coated.

4.   Serve the coleslaw cold as a creamy and crunchy side dish.

3. **Caprese Salad**:

- Ingredients:

    - Fresh mozzarella cheese, sliced

    - Tomatoes, sliced

    - Fresh basil leaves

    - Balsamic glaze (or balsamic vinegar and honey)

    - Extra virgin olive oil

    - Salt and pepper

- Instructions:

1.   Arrange alternating slices of fresh mozzarella cheese and tomatoes on a serving platter.

2.   Tuck fresh basil leaves between the cheese and tomato slices.

3.   Drizzle with balsamic glaze and extra virgin olive oil.

4.   Season with salt and pepper to taste.

5.   Serve the Caprese salad cold as a simple yet elegant side dish.

These affordable side salads with simple dressings are not only quick and easy to prepare but also offer a refreshing contrast to richer main dishes, adding color, texture, and flavor to your meal.

Quick and Easy Grains and Legumes

Grains and legumes are nutritious and versatile ingredients that can be transformed into a variety of budget-friendly side dishes. Here are some ideas for quick and easy grains and legumes:

1. **Quinoa Salad**:

    - Ingredients:

        - Cooked quinoa

        - Assorted vegetables (such as bell peppers, cucumber, cherry tomatoes, and avocado), diced

        - Fresh herbs (such as parsley, cilantro, or mint), chopped

        - Lemon vinaigrette dressing (lemon juice, olive oil, Dijon mustard, salt, and pepper)

    - Instructions:

1.   In a large bowl, combine cooked quinoa, diced vegetables, and chopped fresh herbs.

2.   Drizzle with lemon vinaigrette dressing and toss until evenly coated.

3.   Serve the quinoa salad cold as a protein-packed and flavorful side dish.

2. **Black Bean Salad**:

- Ingredients:

    - Canned black beans, drained and rinsed

    - Corn kernels (fresh, frozen, or canned)

    - Red bell pepper, diced

    - Red onion, diced

    - Fresh cilantro, chopped

    - Lime vinaigrette dressing (lime juice, olive oil, honey, salt, and pepper)

- Instructions:

1.   In a large bowl, combine canned black beans, corn kernels, diced red bell pepper, diced red onion, and chopped fresh cilantro.

2.   Drizzle with lime vinaigrette dressing and toss until evenly coated.

3.   Serve the black bean salad cold as a zesty and satisfying side dish.

3. **Brown Rice Pilaf**:

- Ingredients:
    - Cooked brown rice
    - Onion, diced
    - Garlic, minced
    - Frozen mixed vegetables (such as peas, carrots, and corn)
    - Olive oil
    - Soy sauce
    - Sesame oil (optional)
- Instructions:

1.   In a large skillet or wok, heat olive oil over medium heat.

2.   Add diced onion and minced garlic to the skillet and cook until softened.

3.   Stir in frozen mixed vegetables and cook until heated through.

4.   Add cooked brown rice to the skillet and drizzle with soy sauce and sesame oil (if using).

5.   Stir-fry everything together until well combined and heated through.

6.   Serve the brown rice pilaf hot as a hearty and flavorful side dish.

These quick and easy grains and legumes side dishes are not only nutritious and satisfying but also versatile, allowing you to use up leftover ingredients and customize them to suit your taste preferences.

Desserts don't have to break the bank to be delicious and satisfying. With a bit of creativity and smart shopping, you can enjoy sweet treats without overspending. In this section, we explore low-cost dessert ideas that are both budget-friendly and indulgent.

Budget-Friendly Fruit-Based Desserts

Fruits are nature's candy, offering sweetness and natural flavors that can be transformed into delightful desserts without costing a fortune. Here are some ideas for budget-friendly fruit-based desserts:

1. **Mixed Fruit Salad**:

    - Ingredients:

        - Assorted fruits (such as strawberries, blueberries, grapes, kiwi, and oranges), chopped or sliced

        - Fresh mint leaves, chopped (optional)

        - Honey or maple syrup (optional)

    - Instructions:

1. In a large bowl, combine chopped or sliced fruits.

2.   Sprinkle with chopped fresh mint leaves (if using) for added flavor.

3.   Drizzle with honey or maple syrup (if desired) for extra sweetness.

4.   Toss until evenly coated and serve the mixed fruit salad cold as a refreshing and nutritious dessert.

2. **Fruit Parfait**:

- Ingredients:

    - Greek yogurt

    - Assorted fruits (such as berries, sliced bananas, and diced mango)

    - Granola or crushed graham crackers

- Instructions:

1.   In serving glasses or bowls, layer Greek yogurt with assorted fruits and granola or crushed graham crackers.

2.   Repeat the layers until the glasses or bowls are filled.

3.   Serve the fruit parfait immediately as a light and satisfying dessert.

3. **Grilled Fruit Skewers**:

- Ingredients:

- Assorted fruits (such as pineapple chunks, peach slices, and strawberry halves)

- Wooden skewers

- Honey (optional)

- Cinnamon (optional)

- Instructions:

1. Preheat a grill or grill pan over medium heat.

2. Thread assorted fruits onto wooden skewers, alternating different types of fruit.

3. Grill the fruit skewers for 2-3 minutes on each side, or until grill marks appear and the fruit is softened.

4. Drizzle with honey and sprinkle with cinnamon (if desired) for extra flavor.

5. Serve the grilled fruit skewers hot as a delicious and healthy dessert.

These budget-friendly fruit-based desserts are not only simple to prepare but also packed with vitamins, minerals, and antioxidants, making them a guilt-free indulgence for any occasion.

Affordable Baked Treats with Pantry Staples

Baking your own treats at home is not only cost-effective but also allows you to customize flavors and ingredients to suit your taste preferences. Here are some ideas for affordable baked treats using pantry staples:

1. **Classic Chocolate Chip Cookies**:

    - Ingredients:

        - All-purpose flour

        - Granulated sugar

        - Brown sugar

        - Butter

        - Eggs

        - Vanilla extract

        - Baking soda

        - Salt

        - Chocolate chips

    - Instructions:

1.   Preheat the oven to 375°F (190°C).

2.   In a large mixing bowl, cream together butter, granulated sugar, and brown sugar until light and fluffy.

3.	Beat in eggs and vanilla extract until well combined.

4.	In a separate bowl, whisk together all-purpose flour, baking soda, and salt.

5.	Gradually add the dry ingredients to the wet ingredients, mixing until just combined.

6.	Stir in chocolate chips until evenly distributed throughout the dough.

7.	Drop rounded tablespoons of dough onto baking sheets lined with parchment paper.

8.	Bake in the preheated oven for 8-10 minutes, or until golden brown around the edges.

9.	Allow the cookies to cool on the baking sheets for a few minutes before transferring them to wire racks to cool completely.

2. **Banana Bread**:

- Ingredients:

  - Ripe bananas, mashed

  - All-purpose flour

  - Granulated sugar

  - Butter or vegetable oil

- Eggs

- Baking soda

- Salt

- Optional mix-ins (such as chopped nuts or chocolate chips)

- Instructions:

1. Preheat the oven to 350°F (175°C).

2. In a large mixing bowl, cream together mashed bananas, granulated sugar, and softened butter or vegetable oil.

3. Beat in eggs until well combined.

4. In a separate bowl, whisk together all-purpose flour, baking soda, and salt.

5. Gradually add the dry ingredients to the wet ingredients, mixing until just combined.

6. Fold in optional mix-ins such as chopped nuts or chocolate chips.

7. Pour the batter into a greased loaf pan.

8. Bake in the preheated oven for 50-60 minutes, or until a toothpick inserted into the center comes out clean.

9.   Allow the banana bread to cool in the pan for 10 minutes before transferring it to a wire rack to cool completely.

3. **Simple Brownies**:

- Ingredients:

  - All-purpose flour

  - Granulated sugar

  - Cocoa powder

  - Butter

  - Eggs

  - Vanilla extract

  - Baking powder

  - Salt

- Instructions:

1.   Preheat the oven to 350°F (175°C).

2.   In a saucepan, melt butter over low heat.

3.   Remove the melted butter from heat and stir in granulated sugar, cocoa powder, eggs, and vanilla extract until well combined.

4.   In a separate bowl, whisk together all-purpose flour, baking powder, and salt.

5.   Gradually add the dry ingredients to the wet ingredients, mixing until just combined.

6.   Pour the batter into a greased baking dish.

7.   Bake in the preheated oven for 20-25 minutes, or until a toothpick inserted into the center comes out with a few moist crumbs.

8.   Allow the brownies to cool in the baking dish before cutting them into squares.

These affordable baked treats with pantry staples are not only comforting and delicious but also easy to make, making them perfect for satisfying your sweet tooth without breaking the bank.

DIY Frozen Treats for Hot Days

Homemade frozen treats are a fun and economical way to beat the heat while satisfying your sweet cravings. Here are some ideas for DIY frozen treats for hot days:

1. **Frozen Fruit Pops**:

   - Ingredients:

     - Assorted fruits (such as berries, kiwi, and mango), chopped or sliced

- Fruit juice or coconut water

- Honey or agave syrup (optional)

- Instructions:

1.   Fill popsicle molds with chopped or sliced fruits, leaving some space at the top.

2.   Pour fruit juice or coconut water into the molds, covering the fruits.

3.   If desired, drizzle with honey or agave syrup for extra sweetness.

4.   Insert popsicle sticks into the molds and freeze until solid.

5.   Once frozen, remove the fruit pops from the molds and enjoy them as a refreshing and healthy frozen treat.

2. **Homemade Frozen Yogurt**:

- Ingredients:

  - Greek yogurt

  - Honey or maple syrup

  - Vanilla extract

  - Assorted mix-ins (such as fresh fruit, chocolate chips, or chopped nuts)

- Instructions:

1. In a mixing bowl, combine Greek yogurt, honey or maple syrup, and vanilla extract to taste.

2. Stir in assorted mix-ins such as fresh fruit, chocolate chips, or chopped nuts.

3. Pour the mixture into a shallow dish and spread it out evenly.

4. Freeze the yogurt mixture for 2-3 hours, stirring every 30 minutes to break up any ice crystals and maintain a creamy texture.

5. Once frozen, scoop the homemade frozen yogurt into bowls or cones and enjoy it as a creamy and refreshing treat.

3. **DIY Ice Cream Sandwiches**:

- Ingredients:
    - Chocolate chip cookies or graham crackers
    - Ice cream of your choice
    - Optional toppings (such as sprinkles or chopped nuts)
- Instructions:

1. Place a scoop of ice cream between two chocolate chip cookies or graham crackers to form a sandwich.

2.   If desired, roll the edges of the ice cream sandwich in optional toppings such as sprinkles or chopped nuts.

3.   Wrap each ice cream sandwich individually in plastic wrap and freeze until firm.

4.   Once frozen, unwrap the ice cream sandwiches and enjoy them as a nostalgic and satisfying frozen treat.

These DIY frozen treats for hot days are not only fun to make but also customizable, allowing you to experiment with different flavors and ingredients to create your own unique frozen delights.

CHAPTER EIGHT

Budget-Friendly Beverages

Staying hydrated doesn't have to be costly. With a bit of creativity, you can craft refreshing and flavorful beverages without breaking the bank. In this section, we explore budget-friendly beverage ideas that are both economical and satisfying.

Infused Water Varieties Using Inexpensive Ingredients

Infused water is a refreshing and hydrating option that allows you to add natural flavors to your drink without added sugars or artificial ingredients. Here are some ideas for infused water varieties using inexpensive ingredients:

1. **Cucumber and Mint Infused Water**:

    - Ingredients:

        - Cucumber, thinly sliced

        - Fresh mint leaves

        - Water

    - Instructions:

1.   Place thinly sliced cucumber and fresh mint leaves in a pitcher.

2.   Fill the pitcher with water.

3.   Refrigerate for at least 2 hours to allow the flavors to infuse.

4.   Serve the cucumber and mint infused water cold over ice for a refreshing and cooling drink.

2. **Citrus Infused Water**:

- Ingredients:

    - Lemon, thinly sliced

    - Lime, thinly sliced

    - Orange, thinly sliced

    - Water

- Instructions:

1.   Place thinly sliced lemon, lime, and orange in a pitcher.

2.   Fill the pitcher with water.

3.   Refrigerate for at least 2 hours to allow the flavors to infuse.

4.   Serve the citrus infused water cold over ice for a zesty and revitalizing drink.

3. **Berry and Basil Infused Water**:

- Ingredients:

    - Assorted berries (such as strawberries, blueberries, and raspberries)

- Fresh basil leaves

- Water

- Instructions:

1. Place assorted berries and fresh basil leaves in a pitcher.

2. Fill the pitcher with water.

3. Refrigerate for at least 2 hours to allow the flavors to infuse.

4. Serve the berry and basil infused water cold over ice for a burst of fruity and herbaceous flavor.

These infused water varieties using inexpensive ingredients are not only hydrating and refreshing but also customizable, allowing you to mix and match flavors to suit your taste preferences.

Budget-Friendly Smoothie and Shake Recipes

Smoothies and shakes are nutritious and filling beverages that can be customized with affordable ingredients to suit your taste and budget. Here are some ideas for budget-friendly smoothie and shake recipes:

1. **Banana Peanut Butter Smoothie**:

   - Ingredients:

     - Ripe bananas

     - Peanut butter

- Milk (dairy or plant-based)

- Honey or maple syrup (optional)

- Ice cubes

- Instructions:

1. In a blender, combine ripe bananas, peanut butter, milk, and honey or maple syrup (if desired).

2. Blend until smooth and creamy.

3. Add ice cubes and blend again until the desired consistency is reached.

4. Serve the banana peanut butter smoothie cold for a satisfying and protein-packed beverage.

2. **Mixed Berry Yogurt Smoothie**:

- Ingredients:

    - Assorted berries (such as strawberries, blueberries, and raspberries)

    - Greek yogurt

    - Milk (dairy or plant-based)

    - Honey or maple syrup (optional)

    - Ice cubes

- Instructions:

1.   In a blender, combine assorted berries, Greek yogurt, milk, and honey or maple syrup (if desired).

2.   Blend until smooth and creamy.

3.   Add ice cubes and blend again until the desired consistency is reached.

4.   Serve the mixed berry yogurt smoothie cold for a refreshing and nutrient-rich beverage.

3. **Chocolate Banana Shake**:

- Ingredients:
    - Ripe bananas
    - Cocoa powder
    - Milk (dairy or plant-based)
    - Honey or maple syrup (optional)
    - Ice cubes
- Instructions:

1.   In a blender, combine ripe bananas, cocoa powder, milk, and honey or maple syrup (if desired).

2.   Blend until smooth and creamy.

3.   Add ice cubes and blend again until the desired consistency is reached.

4.   Serve the chocolate banana shake cold for a decadent and satisfying treat.

These budget-friendly smoothie and shake recipes are not only delicious and nutritious but also versatile, allowing you to use up ingredients you already have on hand to create tasty and filling beverages.

Simple and Affordable Herbal Tea Blends

Herbal teas offer a soothing and comforting option for hydration, and they can be easily customized with inexpensive ingredients. Here are some ideas for simple and affordable herbal tea blends:

1. **Mint Tea**:

- Ingredients:

    - Fresh mint leaves (or dried mint leaves)

    - Water

- Instructions:

1.   Bring water to a boil in a saucepan.

2.   Remove the saucepan from heat and add fresh mint leaves.

3.   Cover the saucepan and let the mint leaves steep for 5-10 minutes.

4.   Strain the mint leaves and pour the tea into cups.

5.   Serve the mint tea hot or cold for a refreshing and invigorating beverage.

2. **Ginger Lemon Tea**:

- Ingredients:
  - Fresh ginger, sliced
  - Lemon slices
  - Water
- Instructions:

1.   Bring water to a boil in a saucepan.

2.   Add fresh ginger slices and lemon slices to the boiling water.

3.   Reduce the heat and let the tea simmer for 10-15 minutes.

4.   Strain the ginger and lemon slices and pour the tea into cups.

5.   Serve the ginger lemon tea hot or cold for a soothing and warming drink.

3. **Chamomile Lavender Tea**:

- Ingredients:
  - Chamomile flowers (dried or fresh)

- Lavender buds (dried or fresh)

- Water

- Instructions:

1. Bring water to a boil in a saucepan.

2. Add chamomile flowers and lavender buds to the boiling water.

3. Cover the saucepan and let the herbs steep for 5-10 minutes.

4. Strain the chamomile and lavender and pour the tea into cups.

5. Serve the chamomile lavender tea hot or cold for a calming and relaxing beverage.

These simple and affordable herbal tea blends are not only soothing and aromatic but also provide various health benefits, making them an excellent choice for any time of the day.

CHAPTER NINE

Maximizing Your Budget with Meal Prep

Meal prep is a powerful tool for saving time, money, and effort while still enjoying delicious and nutritious meals throughout the week. By strategically planning and preparing meals in advance, you can maximize your budget and minimize food waste. In this section, we'll explore various meal prep strategies aimed at helping you make the most of your resources.

Budget-Friendly Meal Planning Strategies

Effective meal planning is the cornerstone of successful meal prep on a budget. By carefully planning your meals for the week ahead, you can streamline your grocery shopping, reduce impulse purchases, and make the most of ingredients you already have on hand. Here are some budget-friendly meal planning strategies to consider:

1. **Create a Weekly Meal Plan**: Take some time at the beginning of each week to plan out your meals for the upcoming days. Consider factors such as your schedule, dietary preferences, and ingredients you already have in your pantry. Aim for a balance of proteins, carbohydrates, and vegetables to ensure well-rounded and satisfying meals.

2. **Shop Your Pantry and Fridge First**: Before heading to the grocery store, take inventory of what you already have in

your pantry, fridge, and freezer. Incorporate these ingredients into your meal plan to avoid buying duplicate items and reduce food waste.

3. **Choose Budget-Friendly Ingredients**: Opt for affordable staples such as beans, lentils, rice, pasta, and seasonal vegetables when planning your meals. These ingredients are not only cost-effective but also versatile and nutritious, allowing you to create a variety of dishes without breaking the bank.

4. **Plan for Leftovers**: Embrace leftovers as a valuable resource in your meal planning arsenal. Cook larger batches of meals that can be enjoyed as leftovers for lunch or dinner throughout the week. This not only saves time but also reduces the need to cook multiple meals from scratch.

5. **Use Coupons and Discounts**: Keep an eye out for sales, coupons, and discounts on groceries to stretch your budget even further. Take advantage of store loyalty programs, digital coupons, and weekly specials to save money on staple items and ingredients for your meal prep.

By implementing these budget-friendly meal planning strategies, you can streamline your grocery shopping, make the most of your ingredients, and minimize food waste, all while staying within your budget.

Batch Cooking Tips for Saving Time and Money

Batch cooking is a meal prep technique that involves preparing large quantities of food at once and portioning it out for future meals. Not only does batch cooking save time and effort, but it also helps you make the most of your ingredients and minimize food waste. Here are some batch cooking tips for saving time and money:

1. **Choose Recipes That Freeze Well**: When planning your batch cooking sessions, focus on recipes that freeze well and can be reheated easily. Soups, stews, casseroles, and pasta sauces are all excellent options for batch cooking, as they retain their flavor and texture when frozen and reheated.

2. **Invest in Quality Storage Containers**: Invest in a set of high-quality, reusable storage containers in various sizes to store your batch-cooked meals. Opt for containers that are freezer-safe, microwave-safe, and dishwasher-safe for added convenience. Glass containers are durable and environmentally friendly, while plastic containers are lightweight and affordable.

3. **Label and Date Your Meals**: To avoid confusion and ensure that your batch-cooked meals stay fresh, be sure to label and date each container before placing it in the freezer. Use waterproof labels and permanent markers to clearly identify

the contents and date of preparation. This will make it easier to keep track of your inventory and prevent food waste.

4. **Rotate Your Stock**: Rotate your batch-cooked meals regularly to ensure that older items are used up before newer ones. As you prepare fresh batches of meals, move older containers to the front of the freezer to ensure that nothing gets forgotten or lost in the depths of the freezer.

5. **Plan Your Thawing and Reheating Process**: When it comes time to enjoy your batch-cooked meals, plan ahead to thaw them safely and reheat them properly. Thaw frozen meals in the refrigerator overnight or use the defrost setting on your microwave for quicker thawing. Reheat meals thoroughly in the microwave, oven, or stovetop until they reach an internal temperature of 165°F (74°C) to ensure food safety.

By following these batch cooking tips, you can save time, money, and effort while still enjoying delicious and nutritious meals throughout the week.

Freezing and Repurposing Leftovers to Minimize Waste

Minimizing food waste is a key aspect of successful meal prep on a budget. By freezing leftovers and repurposing ingredients, you can make the most of your resources and reduce the amount of food that ends up in the trash. Here are some tips for freezing and repurposing leftovers to minimize waste:

1. **Properly Store Leftovers**: When you have leftover food that you won't be able to eat right away, be sure to store it properly to maintain its freshness and flavor. Transfer leftovers to airtight containers or resealable bags and label them with the contents and date of preparation before placing them in the refrigerator or freezer.

2. **Freeze Individual Portions**: To make it easier to thaw and reheat leftovers as needed, consider portioning them out into individual servings before freezing. This allows you to thaw only what you need and avoid waste. Use freezer-safe containers or portion-sized bags for convenient storage.

3. **Repurpose Leftovers Into New Meals**: Get creative with repurposing leftovers into new meals to prevent boredom and maximize their potential. For example, leftover roasted vegetables can be added to omelets, salads, or grain bowls, while cooked grains can be turned into fried rice or grain-based salads. Use leftover meat or poultry to make sandwiches, wraps, or stir-fries for quick and easy meals.

4. **Keep a "Leftovers Night"**: Dedicate one night per week to enjoying leftovers for dinner. Use this opportunity to clean out the fridge and freezer and prevent food from going to waste. Encourage family members to choose their favorite

leftovers and create their own custom meals for a fun and interactive dining experience.

5. **Compost Food Scraps**: If you have food scraps that aren't suitable for freezing or repurposing, consider composting them instead. Composting is an eco-friendly way to recycle organic waste and create nutrient-rich soil for your garden. Set up a compost bin or pile in your backyard and add fruit and vegetable scraps, coffee grounds, eggshells, and other organic materials to reduce waste and nourish your soil.

By freezing leftovers and repurposing ingredients, you can minimize food waste, save money, and ensure that nothing goes to waste. Get creative in the kitchen and experiment with new recipes and flavor combinations to make the most of your resources and stretch your budget even further.

CHAPTER TEN

Galveston Diet Beyond the Kitchen on a Budget

Living the Galveston Diet lifestyle goes beyond just the food you eat; it encompasses holistic wellness, including physical health, financial well-being, and sustainable lifestyle practices. In this section, we'll explore how you can maintain a Galveston Diet lifestyle while being mindful of your budget and resources.

Affordable Exercise Options for Physical Health

Physical activity is an essential component of the Galveston Diet lifestyle, promoting overall health and well-being. However, gym memberships and fitness classes can be expensive. Here are some affordable exercise options to consider for improving your physical health without breaking the bank:

1. **Walking and Jogging**: Walking and jogging are simple yet effective forms of exercise that require minimal equipment and can be done almost anywhere. Take advantage of local parks, trails, or sidewalks in your neighborhood for free or low-cost outdoor workouts.

2. **Bodyweight Workouts**: Bodyweight exercises such as squats, lunges, push-ups, and planks require no equipment and can be done at home or outdoors. There are plenty of free resources available online, including workout videos and

mobile apps, that provide guidance on bodyweight workouts for all fitness levels.

3. **YouTube Fitness Channels**: Many fitness trainers and enthusiasts share free workout videos on YouTube, covering a wide range of exercise routines, from yoga and Pilates to HIIT (High-Intensity Interval Training) and strength training. Find channels that align with your fitness goals and preferences to access free workout content anytime, anywhere.

4. **Community Recreation Centers**: Check out local community centers or recreation facilities that offer affordable fitness classes, sports leagues, and recreational activities. These programs often provide discounted rates for residents and may offer a variety of options, including swimming, yoga, dance, and more.

5. **Online Fitness Challenges**: Participate in online fitness challenges or virtual events hosted by fitness communities or organizations. These challenges often provide structure, accountability, and community support while being accessible to participants of all fitness levels and budgets.

By incorporating affordable exercise options into your routine, you can prioritize your physical health and well-being without overspending.

Mindful Spending Habits for Long-Term Financial Wellness

Financial wellness is an integral part of the Galveston Diet lifestyle, emphasizing mindful spending habits and responsible financial management. Here are some tips for cultivating long-term financial wellness while living on a budget:

1. **Create a Budget**: Develop a budget that outlines your monthly income, expenses, and savings goals. Allocate funds for essentials such as food, housing, transportation, and healthcare, as well as discretionary spending on non-essential items and activities.

2. **Track Your Spending**: Keep track of your expenses and monitor your spending habits regularly. Use budgeting apps or spreadsheets to categorize your expenditures and identify areas where you can cut back or reallocate funds to align with your financial priorities.

3. **Practice Conscious Consumption**: Adopt a mindful approach to consumption by evaluating your purchases based on their value and alignment with your goals and values. Before making a purchase, ask yourself if it's necessary, if it brings you joy or adds value to your life, and if there are more affordable alternatives available.

4. **Save and Invest Wisely**: Set aside a portion of your income for savings and investments to build financial security and stability over time. Consider opening a savings account, contributing to a retirement plan or investment portfolio, and exploring low-cost investment options such as index funds or robo-advisors.

5. **Avoid Impulse Purchases**: Resist the temptation to make impulse purchases by practicing delayed gratification and mindful decision-making. Take the time to research products, compare prices, and consider alternatives before making a purchase to ensure that it aligns with your budget and financial goals.

By practicing mindful spending habits and prioritizing long-term financial wellness, you can achieve greater financial freedom and security while living the Galveston Diet lifestyle.

Building a Sustainable Galveston Diet Lifestyle on a Budget

Living a sustainable lifestyle is key to the Galveston Diet philosophy, emphasizing environmental stewardship and conscious living. Here are some tips for building a sustainable Galveston Diet lifestyle on a budget:

1. **Reduce, Reuse, Recycle**: Embrace the principles of reduce, reuse, and recycle to minimize waste and conserve

resources. Reduce your consumption of single-use plastics and disposable products, reuse items whenever possible, and recycle materials such as paper, glass, and metal to divert waste from landfills.

2. **Grow Your Own Food**: Consider starting a home garden to grow your own fruits, vegetables, and herbs. Gardening not only allows you to enjoy fresh, organic produce but also reduces your carbon footprint and promotes food self-sufficiency. Choose low-cost or easy-to-grow crops that thrive in your climate and require minimal inputs.

3. **Cook and Eat at Home**: Prepare homemade meals using fresh, seasonal ingredients and minimize food waste by meal planning, batch cooking, and repurposing leftovers. Eating at home not only saves money but also allows you to control the quality and nutritional content of your meals while reducing packaging waste associated with takeout and processed foods.

4. **Conserve Energy and Water**: Practice energy and water conservation habits to reduce your environmental impact and lower utility bills. Turn off lights and appliances when not in use, use energy-efficient lighting and appliances, and fix leaks and drips to conserve water. Consider investing in programmable thermostats, low-flow fixtures, and insulation to improve energy efficiency in your home.

5. **Support Sustainable Practices**: Choose products and services from companies that prioritize sustainability and ethical practices. Look for eco-friendly certifications, such as USDA Organic, Fair Trade, and Forest Stewardship Council (FSC), when shopping for groceries, household goods, and personal care items. Support local businesses and farmers markets to reduce transportation emissions and promote community resilience.

By incorporating sustainable practices into your daily life and making conscious choices that align with your values and budget, you can build a more resilient, environmentally-friendly Galveston Diet lifestyle that benefits both your health and the planet.

CHAPTER 10

31 DAY MEAL PLAN

Here's a varied plan to get you through the month:

Day 1:

- Breakfast: Oatmeal with sliced bananas and a sprinkle of cinnamon.

- Lunch: Black bean and corn salad with a lime vinaigrette.

- Dinner: Baked tilapia fillets with roasted vegetables.

Day 2:

- Breakfast: Scrambled eggs with sautéed bell peppers and onions.

- Lunch: Tuna salad lettuce wraps.

- Dinner: Chicken and vegetable stir-fry with brown rice.

Day 3:

- Breakfast: Greek yogurt with honey and mixed berries.

- Lunch: Lentil soup with a side of whole grain bread.

- Dinner: Baked chicken thighs with mashed sweet potatoes and steamed broccoli.

Day 4:

- Breakfast: Whole grain toast with avocado slices and cherry tomatoes.

- Lunch: Vegetable and bean chili.

- Dinner: Spaghetti squash with marinara sauce and a side salad.

Day 5:

- Breakfast: Smoothie with spinach, banana, and almond milk.

- Lunch: Turkey and cheese whole grain wraps with carrot sticks.

- Dinner: Baked salmon with roasted asparagus and quinoa.

Day 6:

- Breakfast: Overnight oats with peanut butter and sliced apples.

- Lunch: Chickpea salad with cucumber, tomatoes, and feta cheese.

- Dinner: Vegetable curry with brown rice.

Day 7:

- Breakfast: Whole grain pancakes with fresh fruit topping.

- Lunch: Egg salad sandwiches on whole wheat bread.

- Dinner: Baked pork chops with roasted Brussels sprouts and sweet potatoes.

Day 8:

- Breakfast: Breakfast burritos with scrambled eggs, black beans, and salsa wrapped in whole wheat tortillas.

- Lunch: Quinoa salad with diced vegetables and a lemon-tahini dressing.

- Dinner: Baked chicken drumsticks with roasted cauliflower and a side of brown rice.

Day 9:

- Breakfast: Yogurt parfait with granola and sliced peaches.

- Lunch: Veggie-packed minestrone soup with a side of whole grain crackers.

- Dinner: Blackened fish tacos with cabbage slaw and avocado.

Day 10:

- Breakfast: Whole grain toast topped with mashed avocado and poached eggs.

- Lunch: Chickpea and vegetable stir-fry with a teriyaki sauce served over brown rice.

- Dinner: Baked turkey meatballs with marinara sauce, served with zucchini noodles.

Day 11:

- Breakfast: Banana smoothie with spinach, peanut butter, and almond milk.

- Lunch: Quinoa and black bean stuffed bell peppers.

- Dinner: Oven-baked tilapia with lemon herb seasoning, served with roasted vegetables.

Day 12:

- Breakfast: Overnight chia seed pudding with mixed berries.

- Lunch: Lentil and vegetable curry served over brown rice.

- Dinner: Baked chicken thighs with barbecue sauce, roasted sweet potatoes, and green beans.

Day 13:

- Breakfast: Whole grain pancakes with sliced bananas and a drizzle of honey.

- Lunch: Turkey and vegetable stir-fry with a soy ginger glaze, served over quinoa.

- Dinner: Baked cod with a lemon-dill sauce, served with steamed broccoli and couscous.

Day 14:

- Breakfast: Scrambled eggs with sautéed spinach and mushrooms.

- Lunch: Chickpea and avocado salad with a lemon vinaigrette.

- Dinner: Baked pork tenderloin with roasted carrots and mashed potatoes.

Day 15:

- Breakfast: Greek yogurt with honey and chopped walnuts.

- Lunch: Black bean and corn quesadillas with salsa and guacamole.

- Dinner: Oven-roasted chicken breasts with a balsamic glaze, served with roasted Brussels sprouts and quinoa.

Day 16:

- Breakfast: Whole grain toast topped with mashed avocado and sliced tomatoes.

- Lunch: Spinach and feta stuffed chicken breast with a side salad.

- Dinner: Lentil and vegetable stew served with crusty whole grain bread.

Day 17:

- Breakfast: Banana oatmeal pancakes topped with Greek yogurt and berries.

- Lunch: Quinoa and black bean salad with diced bell peppers and a lime vinaigrette.

- Dinner: Baked salmon fillets with roasted asparagus and wild rice.

Day 18:

- Breakfast: Scrambled eggs with sautéed spinach and whole grain toast.

- Lunch: Turkey and vegetable stir-fry with teriyaki sauce served over brown rice.

- Dinner: Baked chicken drumsticks with barbecue sauce, roasted sweet potatoes, and green beans.

Day 19:

- Breakfast: Greek yogurt parfait with granola and sliced strawberries.

- Lunch: Vegetable and chickpea curry served over quinoa.

- Dinner: Baked tilapia with lemon and herbs, served with steamed broccoli and couscous.

Day 20:

- Breakfast: Smoothie bowl topped with sliced bananas, shredded coconut, and chia seeds.

- Lunch: Black bean and corn salad with diced tomatoes and avocado.

- Dinner: Turkey meatloaf with roasted carrots and mashed potatoes.

Day 21:

- Breakfast: Whole grain pancakes with mixed berry compote and a dollop of Greek yogurt.

- Lunch: Lentil soup with a side of whole grain crackers.

- Dinner: Baked pork chops with applesauce, roasted Brussels sprouts, and quinoa.

Day 22:

- Breakfast: Overnight oats with almond milk, sliced almonds, and diced peaches.

- Lunch: Chickpea and avocado salad with a lemon-tahini dressing.

- Dinner: Baked chicken thighs with lemon pepper seasoning, roasted sweet potatoes, and green beans.

Day 23:

- Breakfast: Scrambled eggs with diced bell peppers and onions, served with whole grain toast.

- Lunch: Turkey and vegetable stir-fry with a soy ginger glaze, served over brown rice.

- Dinner: Baked cod with a garlic herb butter sauce, served with roasted asparagus and wild rice.

Day 24:

- Breakfast: Greek yogurt with honey and chopped walnuts.

- Lunch: Black bean and corn quesadillas with salsa and guacamole.

- Dinner: Oven-roasted chicken breasts with balsamic glaze, roasted Brussels sprouts, and quinoa.

Day 25:

- Breakfast: Whole grain toast topped with mashed avocado and sliced tomatoes.

- Lunch: Spinach and feta stuffed chicken breast with a side salad.

- Dinner: Lentil and vegetable stew served with crusty whole grain bread.

Day 26:

- Breakfast: Banana oatmeal pancakes topped with Greek yogurt and berries.

- Lunch: Quinoa and black bean salad with diced bell peppers and a lime vinaigrette.

- Dinner: Baked salmon fillets with roasted asparagus and wild rice.

Day 27:

- Breakfast: Scrambled eggs with sautéed spinach and whole grain toast.

- Lunch: Turkey and vegetable stir-fry with teriyaki sauce served over brown rice.

- Dinner: Baked chicken drumsticks with barbecue sauce, roasted sweet potatoes, and green beans.

Day 28:

- Breakfast: Greek yogurt parfait with granola and sliced strawberries.

- Lunch: Vegetable and chickpea curry served over quinoa.

- Dinner: Baked tilapia with lemon and herbs, served with steamed broccoli and couscous.

Day 29:

- Breakfast: Smoothie bowl topped with sliced bananas, shredded coconut, and chia seeds.

- Lunch: Black bean and corn salad with diced tomatoes and avocado.

- Dinner: Turkey meatloaf with roasted carrots and mashed potatoes.

Day 30:

- Breakfast: Whole grain pancakes with mixed berry compote and a dollop of Greek yogurt.

- Lunch: Lentil soup with a side of whole grain crackers.

- Dinner: Baked pork chops with applesauce, roasted Brussels sprouts, and quinoa.

Day 31:

- Breakfast: Overnight oats with almond milk, sliced almonds, and diced peaches.

- Lunch: Chickpea and avocado salad with a lemon-tahini dressing.

- Dinner: Baked chicken thighs with lemon pepper seasoning, roasted sweet potatoes, and green beans.

THE END